# I've lost it!
## an easy diet for a crazy life

## Sarai Henderson

# DEDICATION

I could not have dreamed more than what God has given me,
nor could I have loved more deeply than the love I have received
from my boys (all three of them).

# CONTENTS

# ACKNOWLEDGMENTS

Thanks to my mom Ruth, my husband Jason and my friend Melanie for sharing your recipes with me.

# 1. MY STORY

I wake up every morning, look in the mirror and see what I consider to be an overweight, flabby, post baby tummy that doesn't seem to want to shrink. Unfortunately that "bounce back body" wasn't bestowed upon me, so I have to deal with what I've been given. But dealing with my tummy doesn't mean I have to accept it.

It baffles me how I got to this point since I was an extremely active teenager. I took ballet and contemporary dance classes at least five days a week, sometimes more, and I was always active in a dance company that performed on a regular bases. I got plenty of exercise.

My first weight gain came as a shock when I quit dancing because of a back injury. It must have been my bad eating habits combined with the loss of physical activity and voilá, like magic, I gained 20 pounds very quickly.

I didn't notice it at first, other than the new, larger pants size, but I still didn't think anything of it. I guess since I was young and naïve, it was just going to be a phase and like all things at that age, it would pass and I would be relatively skinny again.

But nothing changed, not until I got pregnant with my first son. That's when things began to balloon out, literally.

I was hungry all the time, so I ate... and ate... and ate. I didn't take into account that what I was eating wasn't very good for me, again bad eating habits. The only thing my eating was helping with was my ever expanding waist line. I gained a total of fifty pounds during that pregnancy. I shudder just thinking about it.

I kept telling myself "it will all come off easy enough. I'll just work out and it will shrink away." I think that was my way of convincing myself that it was ok to eat like a pig. I didn't see the changes in my face and body. Good thing, because I probably would have broken down and cried every time I saw myself in the mirror.

As soon as my son was born twenty-five pounds came off in an instant. I thought to myself, "Wahoo, here it goes." That inkling of hope floated around in my fragile mind. But when days turned into weeks and weeks into months and still there was no change in my weight, I began to lose hope that I could ever change.

I started to wear layers under my clothes to help suck in the fat rolls and hid my insecurities. I didn't go swimming because I didn't want to be caught dead in a swim suit. I put my life on hold because of my weight.

Over the next year and a half my weight fluctuated a few pounds here and there, but no matter what I tried, it pretty much stayed the same. I had succumbed to the weight gain woes and given up on ever feeling good about myself again.

When I became pregnant with my second son the strangest thing happened. I started to lose weight. At first I was concerned about the baby's wellbeing and how my weight loss would affect the baby's growth. My doctor assured me that my son's heart beat was strong and it can be common in the early stages of pregnancy to lose a little weight. As long as I didn't lose too much weight, I wasn't supposed to worry about it.

I made up my mind this time to eat better and to stay more active. I lost a whole pant size and only gained fifteen pounds by the end of my pregnancy. It was a personal achievement. I made myself a promise that I wouldn't let my weight spiral out of control again and I didn't.

Even though my body was a little thinner I didn't feel right on the inside. Something was physically wrong with me. I had daily stomach aches, heart burn, headaches and nausea. I was tired but couldn't sleep.

My doctor couldn't find anything wrong with me. She suggested drinking more water and taking some vitamins to make me feel happier. None of those things made any difference.

I talked to my mom about how I was feeling and aired my frustrations about not knowing what was wrong. But mother knows best and she had a hunch of what was wrong with me right off the bat.

She suggested that I do an internet search for a condition called Candida. Two of my sisters had been diagnosed with it and I was showing the same symptoms. I looked it up and found out that what I had was a real condition.

Candida is a form of yeast. If you let it run rampant through your body it can cause problems like weight gain and in my case, problems with my digestive system. It can be brought on by infections and the overuse of antibiotics without the replenishing of probiotics. I thought back to when my pain and problems started and it coincided with an infection and a harsh antibiotics regiment.

Well it just made sense at that point. The only thing left to do was to take the easy home test to confirm it. Cover your ears kids, I'm about to get a little graphic about spit.

First thing in the morning, before I ate anything, I took a clear glass, filled it with water and spit a nice big wad of saliva into it. The spit was cloudy and within seconds I started to see tentacle like strings starting to reach for the bottom of the glass. After about fifteen minutes there were ten or more tentacles about an inch long waving in the water. Yep, I had Candida and I had it bad.

I checked my source for the test one more time just to be sure of my results. The spit didn't dissipate or rest on the bottom. That meant that there was an abundant amount of yeast in my saliva that wasn't supposed to be there. I made my husband take the test too, just to be on the safe side. His spit dissipated within minutes.

Over the next few days I researched treatments and weighed my options. I came to the conclusion that diet and probiotics were my best bet. With a little help from my mom, who had done a lot of research on Candida diets, I put together a food plan that was going to be tough but I thought I could handle it.

I started my diet in February and within the first week I thought I was going to die. My symptoms got worse and I felt really sick. My mom assured me that it was the "Candida die off" and that I would feel better soon. Within that first week I lost five pounds and after that I started to feel a lot better. I steadily lost a pound or two a week and by mid April I had lost a total of fifteen pounds.

The best part about it was the day I put my wedding dress on and it fit just like the day I got married. I had hit a mile stone and it felt amazing.

I know that my body is not perfect and probably won't be the same ever again, but I can at least feel better about myself and share my success with others.

You don't have to have Candida to lose weight with this diet, all you need is the will to better yourself and a little know how that's healthy and good for the entire family.

# 2. THE RIGHT KIND OF FOODS

It can be tough to pick out foods that are healthy and on your diet, I know this from firsthand experience. When I first started my food regimen I thought to myself, "What do I have left to eat?" I was a carbaholic and had a tough time finding proteins to replace the carbs.

It took me about a week of being really hungry all the time and eating the same thing over and over till I got into a groove and started making meals that were yummy and filling. It's going to be tough from this point on, but stay positive. Good things will come of this.

## Good Foods:

**Proteins.** Try to make Protein the main focus of your meal. It is relatively sugar free and will fill you up and give you energy to burn for the day.

Good sources of protein come from:

- Beef
- Chicken
- Fish
- Eggs
- Cheese
- Nuts

Try to stay away from processed meats, bacon and packaged lunch meats (Fresh deli meats are ok.) They have lots of sugars and chemicals that your body doesn't need.

**Vegetables.** There is a long list of veggies that are really good for you, but during my studies I also found out that there are veggies that should be avoided because they are very starchy, such as Carrots, Potatoes, Corn, Yam, Beets and Peas. It's ok to eat these foods, but of course everything in moderation.

You can eat as much as you want of these Veggies though:

- Asparagus
- Avocado
- Broccoli
- Cauliflower
- Celery
- Cucumber
- Egg Plant
- Garlic
- Onions
- Peppers
- Spinach
- Zucchini

There are many other veggies that you can eat, but the list would go on and on if I mentioned them all. You get the picture though. Try to eat a veggie with every meal. They are packed full vitamins that are good for your health.

**Fruits.** Surprisingly, this is a tricky subject. Fruits are great for you, but they are also high in natural sugars. Although these sugars are better for you then the package of sweet and low that you dump into your coffee, they are still sugars and for the first few weeks you should avoid them until your body has gotten used to your new diet.

In four weeks try these low sugar fruits:

- Apples
- Any kind of berry
- Lemon
- Lime
- Watermelon
- Cantaloupe
- Honeydew
- Peaches
- Guava
- Nectarine
- Papaya

**Grains.** Yes, there are actual grains that you can eat. And you thought you were going to starve.

Try to find grains that are high in fiber and stay away from the one's that are high in carbs and break down into sugars quickly like wheat, oats, rye and barley.

Try substituting these grains:

- Wild Rice

- Brown Rice

- Buckwheat

- Millet

- Amaranth

- Quinoa

- Flax Seed

- Couscous

**Herbs, Spices and Oils.** Use a lot of herbs, spices and oils. They can improve digestion and can contain antioxidants and antifungals, plus they can spice up your bland meals to make them more appealing to the whole family.

## Calorie Intake:

The last tip I have for you is to make sure you're eating enough calories, that's right, you heard me, I said eat calories. Your body needs at least 1500 to 2000 a day on average to function and since you're not taking in a lot of carbs you'll have to fill that void with other foods.

If you eat too little calories your body will go into starvation mode and gain weight because your body is holding on to the fat to survive. If you go on like that for too long your body will start to eat muscle to sustain itself. That's not what we're going for here. We want to be healthy.

So eat, and if you're hungry before a meal, have a snack.

# 3. LETS TALK ABOUT WATER

**Water.** Ah, H2O, what can be said about this liquid that covers 70% of the planet? Well for starters, if you went without water for only a few days you would die. Studies have shown that 75% of all Americans are chronically dehydrated. When was the last time you had a glass of water?

Before I became sick I was what I called a cokeaholic. I drank a coke or two a day and never touched water. Shame on me. Once I started drinking water I found that I felt better, my headaches were less frequent and I had more energy throughout the day. It's amazing what a little refreshing liquid can do for you.

Try to make it a goal to drink eight to ten glasses of water a day. I know what you're thinking, "Holy cow, that's a lot of water!" Well, don't worry. At first you're going to feel a little water logged and probably increase the trips you're taking to the bathroom, but your body will soon regulate itself and you'll go back to a normal schedule.

Another great fact about water is that it helps curb those annoying hunger pains. A lot of the time, people can't distinguish the difference between hunger and thirst, so the next time you're hungry and it's not meal time try drinking a glass of water. See what happens.

**Soda Pop.** I think it's safe to say that most people know that soda is bad for you. It's packed full of caffeine and sugars among other things, and yet we still drink them. I, myself am guilty of this knowledge.

If you're an avid soda drinker this is going to be tough. You're going to have to quit cold turkey. Just the replacement of fizzy drinks with water in itself will probably help you lose a few pounds.

This goes for diet sodas as well. You didn't think you were going to get away with it that easy, did you? A lot of

Americans think that picking up a diet soda instead of a regular one is doing themselves a favor. Yes, there are fewer calories and sugar but its chock full of caffeine, sodium and artificial sweeteners that are made from chemicals.

Play it safe, drink some water.

**Coffee.** Goes along the same lines as soda. It has caffeine and the growing popularity of coffee shops in America have people drinking venté caramel macchiato's among other hard to pronounce sweet coffee drinks. So why don't you have some coffee with your sugar?

If you're going to have a cup of coffee, make it a decaf and keep it at that. Don't add any extra sugars and try not to have more than one cup a day. I hate to reiterate here but moderation people. That's the key.

**Tea.** There are some teas that have caffeine in them, like black tea and green tea. But on the other hand there are a lot of teas that you can drink. Instead of having that morning cup of coffee try some white fen tea.

If that doesn't fit your fancy try one of these:

- Cinnamon Tea

- Clove Tea

- Chamomile Tea

- Peppermint Tea

- Ginger Tea

- Licorice Tea

- Lemongrass Tea

Tea has antifungal properties and can be good for your digestive system. Give it a try. You might actually like it.

**Juice.** Juice is made from fruit, and fruit has sugar. Can you see where I'm going with this? Try to stay clear of fruit juices. Instead, pick up a V8 or even better, you know what I'm going to say, don't you? WATER!

# 4. DOING GOOD THINGS FOR YOURSELF

**Food Diary.** Knowing the impact of what you put in your body helps significantly when trying to lose weight. You might think, "How bad can that burger really be for me?" Well, let me tell you, you're going to be surprised at what you're eating once you really start tracking your intake.

Make a food diary. It doesn't have to be complicated. Get a note book and keep track of what you ate, how much you ate of it, and the carbs and calories that go along with it. If you don't know where to start here's one you can copy.

I've lost it!

## ~My Food Diary~   Mon  Tue  Wed  Thur  Fri  Sat  Sun  Date:

My 8 glasses of water: ☐ ☐ ☐ ☐ ☐ ☐ ☐ ☐

| What I ate | Amount | Calories | Carbs | Note |
|---|---|---|---|---|
|  |  |  |  |  |
|  |  |  |  |  |
|  |  |  |  |  |
|  |  |  |  |  |
|  |  |  |  |  |
|  |  |  |  |  |
|  |  |  |  |  |
|  |  |  |  |  |
|  |  |  |  |  |

How do you think you did today?:   1   2   3   4   5

What foods did you struggle with today?: _____

Notes: _____
_____
_____
_____

**Physical exercise.** As a working mother of two young boys and a student, finding time to exercise can be a difficult task. Some mornings I'll wake up early and work out before I take my shower, but then I find myself falling asleep at the end of the day at the same time as my boys. I don't get that extra time in the evening to be quiet and relax before bed.

I've come to the conclusion that physical activity doesn't mean five hundred crunches and 2 million squats, although that will do it. Physical activity is just getting up and going. Take a walk on your lunch break, or lunges down the hall at work. People might think you look ridiculous, but when you're looking sexy in that little black dress or suit and tie at the office holiday party, who's going to look ridiculous then?

One of my favorite activities is strapping my one year old in the front pack and taking a 3 mile slow walk. That extra weight gets my heart rate going and burns extra calories. I like to refer to my son as my thirty pound tumor in those instances.

The best way to shed those pounds is cardio. Get your heart rate up and keep it up for an extended amount of time. Cardio helps work the fat from the muscle and brings it to the foreground so your body can burn it better.

Toning exercises like crunches and squats or working with weights helps to tone the muscles and make you stronger and leaner.

You need both of these forms of exercise to form that gorgeous body. So say it with me, cardio and toning, cardio and toning.

**Goals.** It's always a good idea to set yourself some goals. You're goals should be realistic but at the same time a challenge so you feel good about yourself when you've reached them.

The first goal I set was fifty whopping pounds. I wanted to be back to my pre-baby weight and I didn't care how. Well guess what, it took me over three years to reach that goal and I'm pretty sure it had a lot to do with the large size of my commitment and that I wasn't on a particular diet and exercise regiment.

Don't tell yourself, "I'm going to lose two pounds in five months." That's a little too easy and to tell you the truth your body can fluctuate those two pounds during the day.

Instead, set a goal of five pounds in two months. It's doable but challenging and can be done on a busy schedule.

Write it down on a sticky note and plaster it to your bathroom mirror or fridge so you can see it every day. It always helps to have a reminder when things aren't feeling so good.

Maybe your goal can be drinking more water. Try to shoot for that eight to ten glasses of H2O that you should be downing at your desk while working. Smaller daily goals are easier to reach and start to rack up when you reach them on a daily basis.

**Support System.** Is there someone losing weight alongside you? Do you have a friend encouraging you along your journey to skinniness? It's important for your mental well being to have a support system.

It can be easy to become discouraged when trying to lose weight. I know, I've been there. You feel like you're never going to feel good about yourself again, you might as well stop trying. Remember, you're not the only one struggling. A little encouragement goes a long way, so recruit a friend and set some goals together.

# 5. RECIPES

So, now that you have read all about what you can and can't eat, take the first step and start living your life healthier.

I have put together a few recipes to jump start your new meal plan and get you on the right track.

Just remember, everything in moderation and drink lots of water. I know you can do it, I have faith in you.

# **Breakfast Burrito**

Here is a great way to start your day off with a protein packed meal. And it's easy too.

- 2 eggs
- 2 Sausage Links
- Sour cream
- Shredded cheese
- Salsa (optional)
- 1 burrito shell

On a skillet, scramble your eggs and brown your sausage on all sides.

When sausage is cooked, chop it into bite sized pieces.

Warm your burrito shell in the microwave for 10 seconds to make it fold better.

Place eggs, sausage, sour cream, cheese and salsa onto shell. Wrap and serve.

# Taco Soup        Serving size: 4

It's not really a soup, but who wants to eat something called taco mush? You can serve warm or cold, by its self or with tortilla chips. It's also good for parties as a dip.

- 1 lbs ground beef
- 1 cup chopped onion
- 1 can tomato sauce
- 1 packet taco seasoning
- 1 packet of ranch dressing mix
- 2 cups shredded cheddar cheese
- 16 oz of sour cream
- Tortilla chips

Heat frying pan to medium heat. Add onion and ground beef to frying pan. Brown ground beef until cooked thoroughly and onions are caramelized. Drain grease from pan. Reduce heat to simmer.

Add tomato sauce, taco seasoning, ranch dressing mix, cheddar cheese and sour cream to frying pan. Mix thoroughly and bring heat back to warm.

# Low Carb Burrito  <u>Serving size: 4</u>

There are very few carbs in a burrito shell. This dish can be customized to your individual taste. Here's how I like to do it to get a protein packed meal.

- 1 lb ground beef
- 1 cup of brown rice
- 2 taco seasoning packets
- Shredded cheddar cheese
- Sour Cream
- Shredded Lettuce
- Diced tomato
- Diced onion
- Large burrito shells

Brown ground beef in a frying pan until meat is thoroughly cooked. Drain grease from pan. Mix in 1 packet of taco seasoning and half a cup of water.

In a rice steamer, add rice, 2 cups water and 1 packet of taco seasoning. Mix and cook until rice is soft.

Shred Cheese and lettuce and dice tomatoes and onions. Heat large burrito shell in the microwave for 10 seconds to make it soft and easier to fold with out breaking.

Set out your smorgasbord, and enjoy.

# **Lumpia**            By: Melanie Inoncillo

A co-worker of mine brought these wonderful wraps into work one day. I loved them so much; I had to make them myself. Enjoy!

- 1 pound ground beef
- 1 pound ground pork
- 2 cloves crushed garlic
- 1 cup minced carrots
- 1 cup peas
- 1 cup corn
- 1 teaspoon ground black pepper
- 1 teaspoon salt
- 1 teaspoon garlic powder
- 30-60 lumpia wrappers
- 1 egg
- 2 cups vegetable oil for frying

Brown ground beef and pork in a wok or skillet until it's fully cooked. Drain grease. Place ground meat into a large mixing bowl and add garlic, carrots, peas, corn, black pepper, salt and garlic powder. Mix well and put in the fridge to cool enough to handle.

Take a lumpia wrap and put one big heaping scoop of the meat mixture near one side of the wrap. Fold both sides over the ends of the filling and roll neatly, keeping the roll tight as you assemble. Moisten the other side of the wrap with a dab of egg to seal the edge.

Heat wok or skillet over medium heat. Add oil to ½ inch depth and heat for five minutes. Slide lumpia carefully into oil, trying not to splash. Fry the rolls for 1 to 2 minutes, until all sides are golden brown. Drain on paper towels and enjoy.

Lumpia can be frozen easily and cooked at a later date. So make a large batch and share with some friends.

# **Pork Chops**   Serving size: 6

I've never been a big pork chop fan, but to tell you the truth, this recipe isn't too bad.

- 6 center-cut pork chops, 1/2" thick
- 1 egg
- 1 cup milk
- 3/4 cup cornflake crumbs
- 1/4 cup fine dry bread crumbs
- 4 teaspoons paprika
- 2 teaspoons oregano
- 3/4 teaspoon chili powder
- 1/2 teaspoon garlic powder
- 1/2 teaspoon black pepper
- 1/8 teaspoon cayenne pepper
- 1/8 teaspoon dry mustard
- 1/2 teaspoon salt

Beat egg with milk. Place chops in milk mixture and let stand for 5 minutes, turning chops once.

Meanwhile, mix together cornflake crumbs, bread crumbs, spices, and salt.

Spray a 9x13-inch baking pan with nonstick spray coating.

Remove chops from milk mixture. Coat thoroughly with crumb mixture.

Place chops in pan and bake in 375º F oven for 20 minutes. Turn chops and bake 15 minutes longer or till no pink remains.

# Roast          By: Jason Henderson

I love having a husband that can cook and is conscious of my dietary needs. He makes a mean roast.

- 3lb beef roast
- 3 cans cream of mushroom soup
- 3 cans beef broth
- 2-3 large onions
- 3-5 red potatoes
- 4 carrots

Cut potatoes, onion and carrots into large bit sized pieces.

Put a scattering of veggies on the bottom of the crock pot. Cover with one can of cream of mushroom soup and one can of beef broth.

Place roast in pot and surround it with the rest of the veggies, soup and broth. Make sure the roast is mostly covered with liquid to keep it moist as it cooks.

Put the lid on the crock pot and cook on high for 8-10 hours.

When roast is done, add a quarter of a cup of flower to the gravy to help thicken.

Serve and enjoy!

# **Parmesan Chicken**

You can add more spices to your crumb mix if you so desire.

- 4 small boneless chicken breasts
- 6-10 Ritz crackers, finely crushed
- ¼ cup parmesan cheese
- 1 egg
- 2 tsp. olive oil

Mix crackers and parmesan cheese in small bowl. Dip chicken breast in egg and roll it in the crumb mixture. Try to evenly coat both sides.

Heat oil in a large skillet on medium heat. Add chicken and cook for 5 to 6 minutes on each side or until golden brown.

# Potato Soup          By: Ruth Fuller

There is no food in the world I love more than potatoes and one of the ways I like to eat them is with some cheese. Yum!!!

- 1lb of potatoes
- 4 cans chicken broth
- Ham, chopped
- Cheddar cheese, shredded
- Parmesan cheese

Peal and cut potatoes into thirds. Put potatoes into a large pot and fill with chicken broth till the potatoes are covered. Boil potatoes until soft. Remove from heat and mash with liquid still in the pot.

Add chopped ham, cheddar cheese and parmesan cheese to the potatoes. Mix well and serve as a meal or a side dish.

# <u>Sugar Free Fruit Desert</u>

This recipe is awesome when you want something sweet but don't want the guilt that comes along with breaking your diet. It can be served by it's self or blended into a fruit smoothie, just add ice.

It's also extremely easy!

- Sugar Free whipped cream
- Fresh or frozen strawberries, blueberries, blackberries and raspberries.

In a large mixing bowl, add all ingredients and stir them together.

I told you it was easy.

# ABOUT THE AUTHOR

Sarai grew up south of Portland, Oregon with her four brothers and three sisters. She danced ballet, contemporary and hip hop for fourteen years before she was forced to quit due to a back injury. She now lives in Portland with her husband and two boys writing and enjoying life.